# "OH, SO THAT IS WHY YOU TALK ABOUT POOP."

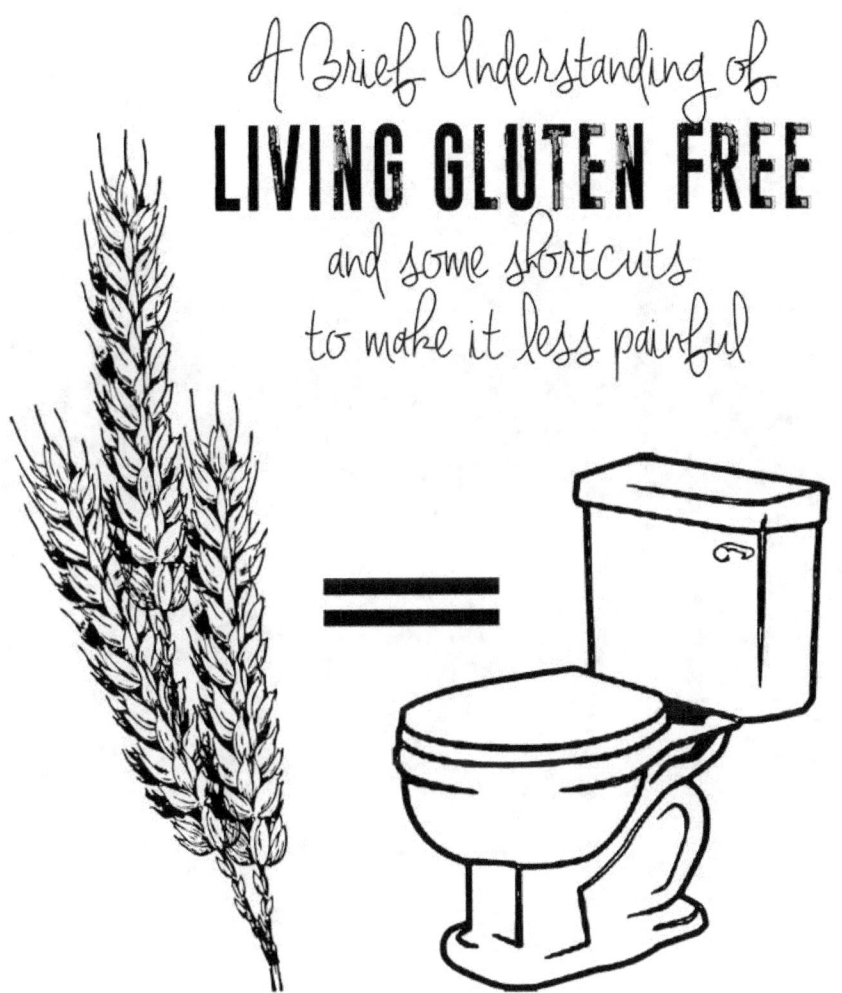

# "OH, SO THAT IS WHY YOU TALK ABOUT POOP."

## THE GLAMOROUS
### YET NOT QUITE APPEALING

*Gluten Free Lifestyle*

**ANDREA YANCY**

" Oh, so that is why you talk about poop."
The Glamorous Yet Not Quite Appealing
Gluten Free Lifestyle
Andrea Yancy

This book is not meant by any means to be a nutrition
or health guide. Consult your doctor before choosing to
try any new medications, diets or lifestyle changes.

Books are available for sale through
several locations. Visit
https://simplysweetandsalty.blogspot.com
For more information.

This book is dedicated to my mom,
for helping me find new ways to approach life;
to my dad,
for being that ray of sunshine on the dreary day;
and also to my brother, Matthew,
for being the comedic relief when I needed it most.

---

"THEREFORE I TELL YOU,
WHATEVER YOU ASK FOR IN PRAYER,
BELIEVE THAT YOU HAVE RECEIVED IT,
AND IT WILL BE YOURS." -MARK 11:24 (NIV)

# CONTENTS

# INTRODUCTION

# PREFACE

This book will be a very real interpretation of how gluten messed me up royally, both inside and out, and how I use the gluten free lifestyle to my advantage. Expect the good, the bad, the ugly, and some crazy stories! Actually, it's better if you don't have any expectations. This book will take you through the many steps from the beginning signs of gluten intolerance, all the way to what I do when I'm glutened, what I eat, and how my family, friends and relationships have changed.

How do you know if this book is something you should read?

If you answer yes, to any of these questions, KEEP READING!

1. Are you gluten intolerant/sensitive or have Celiac Disease?

2. Do you know anyone who has any of the above?

3. Do you have stomach problems and /or are curious about what might help?

4. Do you feel sick after eating?

5. Do you have problems with your bowel movements? (Don't be shy!)

6. Are you bored?

7. Do you like tacos and wine?

8. Do you need some humor in your life?

If you answered yes to any of the questions···
KEEP READING! You won't be sorry!

P.S. I am a huge fan of picture books and will never truly grow up enough to say that pictures aren't my favorite. So, with that confession I'm going to do my best to add some photos, quips, and food hacks. And I'll try to spare you on the gritty bathroom stories that almost anyone going through switching to a gluten free diet understands.

# PREFACE PART 2

## Welcome to the gluten free lifestyle!

If you are new to the gluten free club or even a seasoned veteran, I welcome you into a long, rocky road, that sometimes leads to special treatment! But, often leads to uncomfortable run-ins with hot nurses and random strangers in public restrooms.

If you are not gluten free but are either interested in knowing more for either yourself or someone you know, you have gained **much respect!** Any interest in supporting someone who is gluten free is amazing and much needed support.

This is not an easy road to travel and it is easier when support is there. I however, say with much joy, that I do not regret my decision one bit, as a matter of fact, I couldn't be happier!

Now, for those of you who are reading this book simply because you have nothing else better to do or read... Don't worry, there is enough material in here to make you laugh, that you won't be wasting much time!

Alright, on with the story!

# COUNTING THE MONTHS BEFORE GLUTEN WAS A WORD IN MY VOCABULARY

# MONTH 1

You're probably wondering why I didn't choose the cliché chapter or part 1 for the chapter titles. Let's be honest, if you're going through the changes or know someone who is deciding to be gluten free (whether it's by choice or by the absolutely rotten luck hand you've been dealt) time goes by very slowly and you take it all day by day.

So the story goes...Growing up, my parents were always cooking at home! I never had any food allergies or any problems with health until college actually. I realized one day at a swim meet that I had an allergy to bananas (trust me I still don't understand that one either.) Mom has been allergic to banana for as long as I can remember and I always thought she was just crazy (sorry mom!). I realized that the pain I was feeling after eating a banana was probably one of the worst feelings in the world! My stomach would cramp up and I'd be lying in a ball in the fetal position for several hours, with a completely blown up (or bloated for the meek) stomach. And to make it worse I could not go to the restroom even if I wanted to! This is much unlike how the gluten problems treat me; but that's another story for a bit later in the book. Did I mention there are some details in here that aren't sugar coated? (Even though I love some chocolate coated everything!)

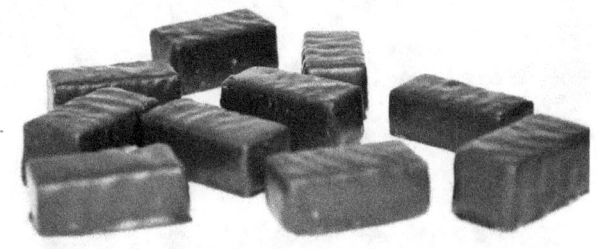

# MONTH 6
## New job and new home

I moved off to the great city of Orlando for college, dorm life, and found a job at the good ole local crab shack. Only a few weeks into the job and I found out I was allergic to shell-fish. I never went into anaphylactic shock, but I did have issues with my throat itching and my face swelling up. It wasn't too glamorous and my coworkers enjoyed looking at "a bug eyed freak" I'm sure. I grew up in Florida and was always considered a southern girl or a beach bum, whichever you choose. All of that being said, I have been eating shrimp, crab, and lobster since I can remember! It's a southern thing that I'm proud to have grown up with, eating those good ole Florida shrimp boils and going to fish fry's! Once I became more allergic to certain foods I did not enjoy the fish fry as much as I used to but I always enjoy the company!

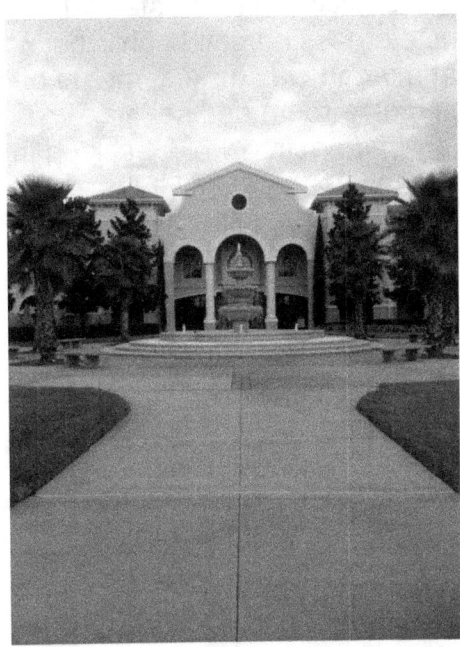

Photo: One of the many images of the beautiful campus I was living on. I wish I could have spent more time enjoying the campus. I however, spent a very large amount of time sitting inside and being sick or sleeping.

# MONTH 9
## Hello hospital folks

I made it about three months into college before my first hospital visit! And no there is no mistake with me using an exclamation point. I'm genuinely impressed that my body held out as long as it did! I was home to visit my family for the weekend and wasn't feeling great as per usual. I don't remember what set it off but I do remember what landed me in the wonderful place with the smell of sterilizer and well... Let's be honest, it smells like a hospital and nothing can quite match it.

Anyways, I was coming out of my room to sit on the couch and watch NCIS with my lovely mother (it was her favorite show and might even still be) and I sat on the edge of the couch (and always get into trouble for doing so!) all of a sudden my head was spinning, I couldn't see straight, I was sweating and I heard a loud BANG. That bang was actually the noise from my head hitting the T.V. stand. I had just experienced a complete passing out. I came back to just enough to realize that my dad was picking me up off the ground to take me to the dining room and set me in a chair. I buckled and hit the ground again. I woke back up in the chair and couldn't hold myself up, focus my eyes, or complete a sentence. On top of the craziness, I was hugging a trash can and being carried to the truck and on my way to the hospital.

I was given an IV, blood tests, and was told that I was dehydrated. Awesome and pointless hospital trip! No real answers to what was happening in my body.

# MONTH 13
## Dorm life... I think?

Living in the dorms was great, except for the fact that the germs were absolutely everywhere. I don't think that I've ever been so sick! As a matter of fact, my roommates and myself passed sickness back and forth more than a fifth of Jack around a campfire.

I was staying away from shell fish, bananas, and sick people just to keep my health a little better than it had been, and I thought that this was normal because it was just a college thing and everyone was sick around me. I had no idea that being so sick so often was actually abnormal.

I spent most of this time at home with family since it was right around December, which meant that all of the hustle and bustle was starting to kick in with all of the holidays around the corner. I was enjoying the Christmas cookies that both my mom and I would bake each year and not to mention all of the goodies and treats that came along with Christmas time!

Speaking of Christmas, I would like to give you an idea of how much I really loved food. I must admit that when I was a bit younger I never really asked for much for Christmas because I was always happy with what I had. I would however, ask my parents for boxes of macaroni and cheese as well as cookies for Christmas. I know, you are probably thinking that I was starved as a kid or deprived of these foods. That is surely not the case! I just loved my macaroni and cheese. So, imagine my surprise when I started to feel sick after eating it! I also never expected my Christmas list to Santa to change from Macaroni and Cheese to gluten free packaged items that I just can't seem to afford without making six digits and pulling out a second mortgage!

I mentioned all of the food I stayed away from however, I have not yet mentioned that I chose to replace those foods with modified tacos! It started with a simple little taco stand in the back of a convenience store. It escalated into myself trying to make those tacos at home. And eventually, I started turning anything and everything into tacos! When I say anything and everything, I am not exaggerating! BBQ meatball tacos, fruit tacos, chocolate and ice cream filled tacos, turkey sandwich tacos and so many other weird and random combinations that looking back make me smile and will make my roommates cringe.

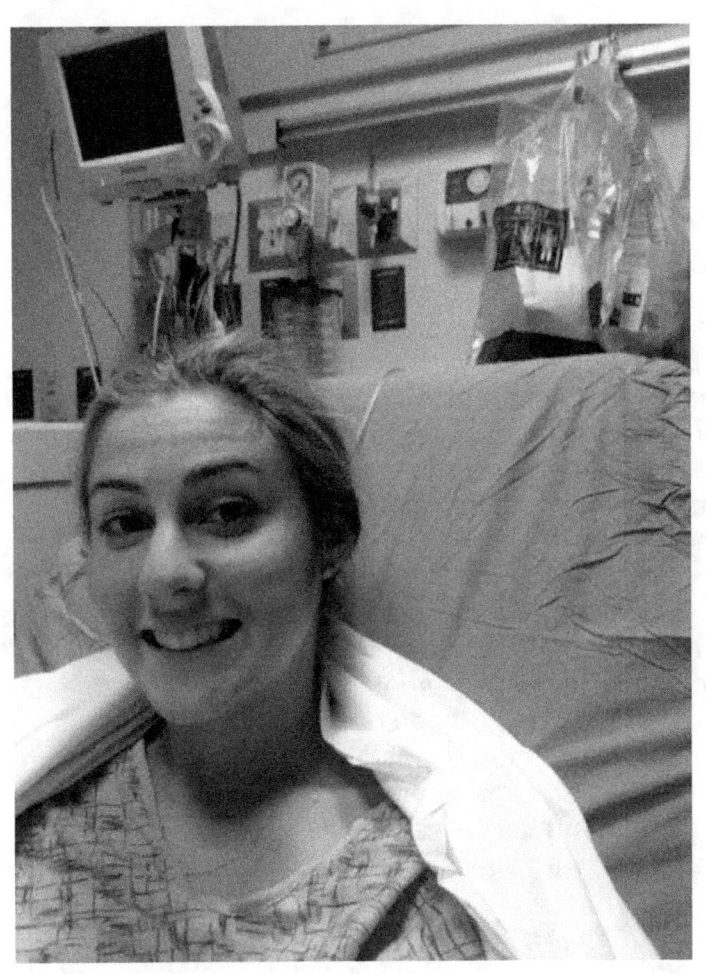

# MONTH 21
## Still sick

I'm a little over a year into living in the city, enjoying the dorm life and going to school. I've had one more hospital visit with the same conclusion! This time it started with my getting very cozy and cuddling with not only a toilet but also a trash can or plastic bag or whatever was available. I did the passing out thing again and handled it a bit better. Except for all of the crying I did when I came back from being passed out (even though I was still delirious), and realized that, when I passed out I woke up enough to throw up into the toilet but I really needed to be sitting on it at the same time.

I was embarrassed beyond all belief because I had just ruined a perfectly good pair of (probably even matching) underwear! I should have been able to get myself off the ground and change but, I could not move and could not think straight. Next thing I knew, I had my roommates helping to change my clothes, call my family, and carrying me to the car on the road again to the lovely IV bag that I was so looking forward to seeing!

For the record, seeing an IV bag used to scare me to death! Anymore, it's like walking into middle school after a long summer off and seeing your best friend. All you want to do is run up and hug them. Well, that is the strong bond that I now feel with that wonderful pouch that seems to be sucked dry in less than an hour! Even with all of this change in pace, I was in pain, yet still thought that I was okay and this was normal. The doctors contributed this trip to one of the following or even a combination of them.

A. Food poisoning from one of those darn frozen meals
B. Too many chocolate chip cookies (I had eaten a dozen that day)
C. Pure exhaustion and dehydration
D. Unexplained causes

What is even more interesting to me about this whole deal is that I was completely blind to everything going on. I ignored the signs of something being absolutely wrong. I started to embrace the fact that I would be sick every other week or so. Making plans became a thing of the past because I never knew if I would be sick or not. Even when I would make plans, I bailed on them well over 80 percent of the time! Looking back, I was actually a miserable person to be around and I feel insanely terrible for everyone who was there and helped me when I was sick (a million times).

Another funny random thought is about the school health care. I had been visiting the school nurses more often than I would come home to see my family! (I was actually home almost every other week, so maybe about the same amount that I had seen them.) I was visiting them for the coughs, sneezes, head aches, sore throats, nausea, aches and pain everywhere, and so many other random symptoms I could not even express to you. (Not to mention, I would go visit the lovely nurses with my roommates when they were sick with Mono or whatever other heebie jeebie contagion they or myself had.)

# MONTH 25
## Confession Time

Are you bored yet with these stories? I am. This one is the same story all over again. Another evening passing out, being carried, delirious statements, needles in my arm, and no answers. Now, time for some humor!

*Did I mention some of the craziest things I have said after*

*passing out and still delirious?*

## WHAT I SAID   VS.   WHAT WAS IN MY MIND

| | |
|---|---|
| " Hey mom, did you see his tattoo? He has a tattoo! He's hot!" | Talking about a male nurse whom I don't even know if I saw him through non-blurry and dazed eyes. |
| " OH NO! My under garments don't match! What if they see that they don't match!? Bre and Simone (two of my friends from way back) always said they should match in case of a hot fireman or doctor!" | This was just ridiculous and I still laugh about it. I actually may never ever live this one down. |
| " I want grapes and sprite. Can we have grapes and sprite when I get home?" | I seriously wanted grapes and sprite because I was so dehydrated and hungry! |
| " IT COULD BE WORSE!" | This is one of my always go-to lines! |

# VEGETABLE SOUP RECIPE

I would like to say that during these few months of feeling terrible, I became a professional at making soups. I made soup out of everything and if I didn't make it myself, rest assured that soup was the only thing I was buying when I ate out or went to the store and didn't feel good enough to cook. How about I just share my favorite soup recipe so you can try it out yourself!

## Ingredients

Consomme - Onions

Potatoes - Celery

Carrots - Broccoli

Green Beans - Corn

Salt - Pepper

## Instructions

Throw everything into one pot and season as you so choose. **Cook for about 20 minutes on the stove!**

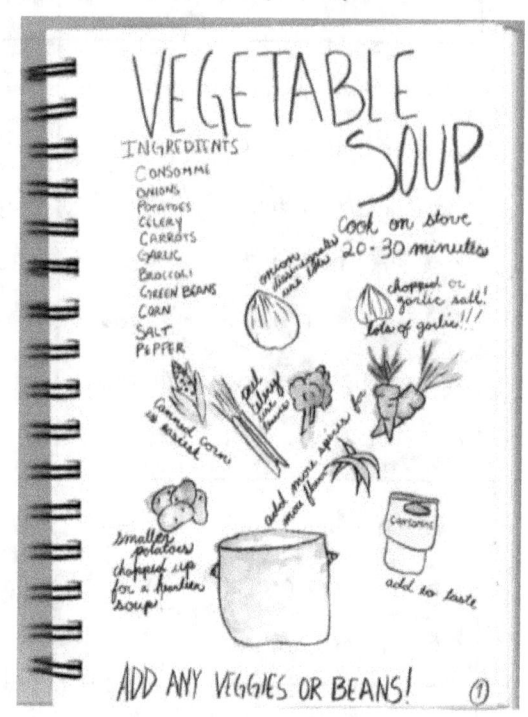

### Easiest soup ever!

I will say that the recipe on here is the most vague recipe ever only because I have changed the ingredients so many times. I enjoy adding in thyme, rosemary, rice noodles, potatoes, lots of garlic, and sometimes beans. I never really had a set recipe for this because it is similar to a 'dump' soup. Whatever is in the kitchen is what I used for the soup.

# GLUTEN
# AND HOW I KNOW IT TODAY

# WHAT IS GLUTEN?

Gluten is a protein found in wheat, rye and barley as well as a myriad of products and it's something that the body has a difficult time digesting.

Eating gluten free is still a topic that many people are not quite accustomed to yet. Honestly, most people do not even know what it is or why some of us can not eat it. All of that being said, allow me to simply explain what Celiac Disease is. When someone with Celiac Disease ingests any amount of gluten it damages the villi (think of these as little nutrient absorbing cushions) in their small intestine. The ingestion of gluten creates an alert for their immune system to attack which flattens out the villi. When the villi are damaged, nutrients are not being absorbed as they should be and continuing to eat gluten can cause other health problems down the road. Celiac Disease is an autoimmune disorder that is actually hereditary and is passed down through the family. Now, for those of us who are not diagnosed with Celiac Disease there are two other types of sensitivity that shows the same symptoms. These are known as Non-Celiac Gluten Sensitivity and Non-Celiac Wheat Sensitivity. All three of these are serious matters and can affect someone's health drastically.

When I first heard of gluten I thought it meant only wheat products. I have never been so sadly mistaken. As a matter of a fact, allow me to expose some of the expected as well as some of the sneakiest forms of Gluten I've come across. **TAKE NOTE:** This is a list of most of the gluten filled products we can not eat. However, it does not list them all. **ALWAYS READ THE LABELS!**

MALT ORZO SOUP LUNCH MEAT

LICORICE Beer MATZA SOY SAUCE

Farina PLayDoh

Stamps/Envelopes MUSTARD (ALE) Couscous Oats

Instant Coffee Vitamins/Medicines

Imitation Crab Meat communion Wafers FU

Semolina Bran

Malt Vinegar WHEAT

Shortening Vodka(flavored)

Pies Teriyaki Maida

Triticale ICE CREAM BABY POWDER

STARCH Baking Powder PANKO CRUMBS MIR SPELT

FARRO DEXTRIN (FOUND IN MEDICINE) Kamut

Durrham Maltodextrin Graham Gravy

Bulgar Rye Lotions

Bouillon Cubes Cooking Spray

CARAMEL COLOR Lipstick Chocolate

Tabbouleh BBQ Sauce Sunscreen

Pretzels Nut Mixes KETCHUP Chewing Gum

Barley

CAUTION: READ ALL LABELS

(EVEN ON SAFE ITEMS)

GF

# HOW DO YOU KNOW IF YOU HAVE A GLUTEN INTOLERANCE?

Should I start with the most obnoxious and most obvious examples, or should I be one of the people who shocks you with a painful reality before we get to the examples that you have already experienced, or that your friend/ family/ significant other is complaining about? Yes… I asked you that question hoping there would be an answer but I think I will list off things as they come to my mind instead. Fair enough?

# SIGNS OF GLUTEN INTOLLERANCE

DENTAL/ BONE DISORDERS Constipation
Gas/Bloating WEIGHT LOSS Migraines
BRAIN FOG Eczema
Acid Reflux
Joint Pain Weakness Exhaustion
Mouth Sores Fertility Problems Anxiety
DIARRHEA Depression Anemia

# SO WHY DO I EAT GLUTEN FREE?

I guess I haven't even gotten to the whole gluten factor in my life yet. I was feeling terrible and could not seem to find any sort of relief of my symptoms so, I did research! As we all know, when you do research on any of your symptoms online, and you try to diagnose yourself, almost 100% of the time the internet says you have cancer, go see a doctor. I knew that I was blessed enough to say that this just was not the case, and that is when I decided to visit a homeopathic doctor. To be honest I thought it was the biggest load of crap I've ever heard. However, I was so sick that I almost fainted in his office, I felt dizzy, nauseous, weak and quite frankly, I felt terrible. I was at my wit's end with how terrible I was feeling and I didn't know where else to go, so I gave doc a try. I was tested for innumerable allergies including dust, pollen, wood, poultry, dairy, gluten and i'm not even sure what else. I tested positive for every last one of the allergies. Due to some cool allergy resetting technique, I was retested and cleared for all of the allergies after only a few weeks and short visits. I was also told that I had a bad case of Candida, a nasty parasite that was making me feel nauseous all of the time, and an adrenal deficiency. I don't think that I could have felt any worse especially as bad as I was feeling when I agreed to take almost 20 pills a day. And for the record, I am a big baby when it comes to medicine. I refuse to take any unless I am on death's front door step. That being said, I was taking allergy medicine, Zymex, Dessicated Adrenal and Choline! Whew, that was a mouth full. I think I need a glass of wine after that one!

Finally, Things started to look up! But not too much longer and it would only down spiral worse than it ever had.

# HOW I FOUND OUT THAT GLUTEN HATED ME

I was not aware of what was happening in my body at all.
I was enjoying working out, working a few jobs, playing
sports (swimming, rock climbing and paintball), eating
whatever I wanted whenever I wanted, fishing, and
traveling! It was not until a few months after moving back
home from college, that I realized my health was starting to
dwindle again and rather quickly.

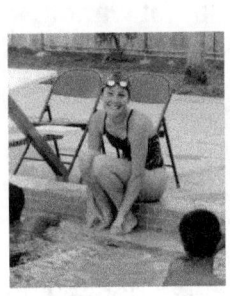 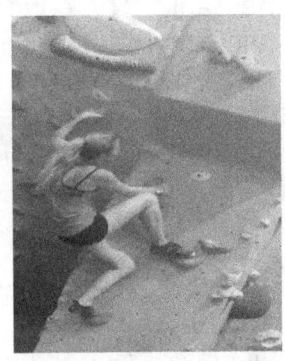 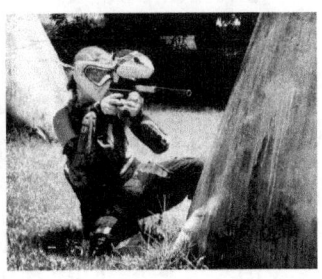

I was introduced to a book called the "Whole 30"
and I was reading the first few pages and became very
quickly intrigued by what I was learning. I learned about
how everything affects your body, and how each thing we
eat digests a different way. I was very much captivated by
the way the body works and I instantly became hooked on
learning more about this meal plan for 30 days. I did all of
the research, I created meal plans, and I started
eliminating things that I could not eat and looking for
alternatives rather than just cutting things out. I was
already down in weight and did not want to lose any more.
I was back on an almost all soup diet again because
everything I ate would make me feel sick. It was time for a
change and this could be my gateway to feeling better!

Allow me to put into perspective how this was already affecting me so that you can understand why I chose to go this route. I had no idea what gluten sensitivity was. I KNEW I was lactose intolerant but never did anything about it. I instead took Lactaid which only helped once per every third or fourth attempt. My parents thought that I had an eating disorder because every time we would sit down for dinner I would eat a few bites and I was running off to the bathroom. I would be hiding in the bathroom for close to an hour some nights and other nights I would be sitting there wishing and praying that I would be able to go to the restroom because maybe it would make the pain a little more bearable. The concern came from several people and I felt like an outcast. I did not want to go out to eat, or even eat anything other than crackers and soup, not only for the pain it would cause, but also for the fear of what else would come into speculation about my health.

Did I mention 'it could have been worse'? (Positivity was a major help going through all of these changes, and this is absolutely my favorite saying and if I was not saying this, I was saying that it was okay because God would have something else planned for me.) I was almost to a breaking point but knew that there was a reason behind everything that I had been going through. I have not had a whole lot of luck with figuring out my health problems but man I still didn't think there was much wrong with me, I thought that this was still going to be okay and that maybe I was just stressed or tired or had something else silly happening.

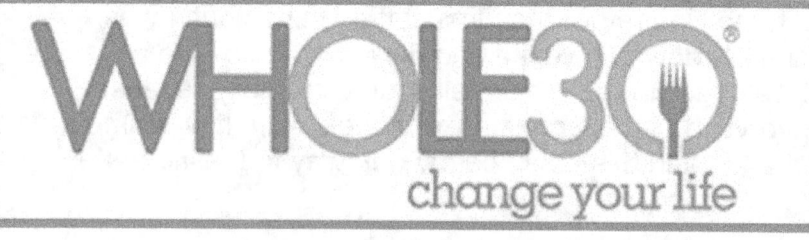

I started the "Whole 30" diet (there is a reference page in the back that you can refer to if you would like to find out more) and it is exactly as they say it is. There were some serious mood swings. I was detoxing my body and I was determined to feel better! For those of you who are not quite sure what the "Whole 30" is, here is a quick idea. It isn't quite a diet. It is more of a detox than anything, and it means that you can not have any Sugar, Dairy, Grains, Legumes or Alcohol. (Quietly sobbing because it counts out wine.)

You are however, allowed to have fruit (still crying because wine is not considered grapes), veggies, meat and healthy fats. Lara bars are on the list of things you are allowed to have... I think I extended this rule a little because I ate SO MANY, I should have just bought stock in the dang company.

I am very excited to say, I started enjoying fruits and veggies much more than I used to. Also, within a week or two of the diet I was still working out and I must say, eating clean was doing me well, not only for how I was feeling but the way that the muscle was building, and I was gaining some weight back! Oh, and I guess I should mention one flaw I encountered during my "Whole 30" I can go ahead and say that my first time reintroducing food was peanut butter and I felt like a slug and was miserable after eating it. I learned that peanuts are something my body doesn't enjoy. This continued and I found that beans, gluten, lactose, and peanuts are ALL things that I just shouldn't eat. I was devastated to learn that my body was revolting against me! I refused to accept those results!

Even after doing this diet I started eating 'cheat' gluten filled meals once a week or so. Every single time I would do it, I would be bent over, or on a toilet, or sleeping on the couch for the rest of the week. It never really struck me that I was not making any sense by doing this. A few months later, my mom and I were on a road trip and I stayed away from all things gluten. As a matter of fact I actually did eat some but I would only take a small bite just to 'taste' whatever my mom's meals were since I was always ordering things not containing gluten.

With myself not feeling good, I was doing some silly things that I just am not proud of at all. For instance, we had some fantastic Beignets from an amazing Cajun style restaurant in South Carolina and because I was so scared of getting sick but wanted to taste them, I chewed on one and spit it out hoping that wouldn't make me sick. I think that was a new low for even me. What I hadn't realized was that I had already been glutened. This meant lots of pain and lots of bathroom visits were coming in the very near future.

What you aren't quite aware of at this point is that, before learning I was intolerant to gluten, I was one of the people who traveled the states in search of the best food! I was eating out multiple times a week, spending all of my money on food and had to scrape up change for the gas money to get there. I was a typical Millennial whose social media was covered in food photos! (I'm slowly getting back to loving food, but more on that later!) I would walk into restaurants that would not even have signs for their building because they were such small town, local restaurants. (Yes I did this in Louisiana and I was scared to death! The food was amazing though! I mean they had lemonade cake and greens! It can't get much better than that, can it?) Basically, my life goal was to eat and travel. And travel in order to eat! My priorities may have been a little off, but I was enjoying it all! I wasn't scared of eating anything and now all of a sudden I am avoiding things that I think make me sick. It actually had gotten so bad that I started to be afraid, annoyed, anxious, and sad when anyone had asked me to go out to dinner. It is one of my favorite things to do and now I am terrified to walk in the building not knowing if I would be able to eat anything or if I would be sick after.

On the last day of the road trip with my mom we were in a hurry to get home because I was not feeling too great. I knew it would take only one small thing to set me into a flare up or allergic reaction or to be honest, I still am not sure what to call the pain I have when I eat something that sets it off. For the purpose of this book let's just call it a Gluten Monster Attack. Since I was worried about eating on the road, my favorite fast food and probably only fast food I will eat even to this day is Wendy's. I ordered a 4 piece chicken nugget because, I thought it would be the safest food I could eat for an upset tummy. Within two hours from the house I was in excruciating pain and I knew right then that it was a wheat problem. I had my mind absolutely set that those chicken nuggets were the LAST gluten filled food I was ever going to eat. And sure enough I have been gluten free since then! Except for those sneaky little gluten monster particles that find their way into my tasty unsuspecting food, and make me feel like I am dying! Hooray!

All of that being said, I went straight to the GF life and never looked back. I did some research on being tested for the gluten intolerance and sensitivity but had to count myself out because, I did not do the testing before I stopped consuming gluten. I also had read how the testing is done! For everyone who has taken the route of being tested for Celiac, gluten intolerance, gluten sensitivity and many other things… You are my role model because, personally, I do not want scopes and probes shoved either down my throat or up my butt. It actually freaks me out just thinking about it! However, if you are Celiac or have any problems you should be doing lots of research and taking care of yourself. This may be the best way to figure out what is really happening inside your body. I would never sway anyone to go one way or another, as long as you are taking care of yourself. I was just too big of a chicken to go get tested and I have said a million and one prayers to thank the good Lord for blessing me with an easy case of the gluten monster attacks. I feel extremely fortunate! This is where we all celebrate because the boring doctor stories, and the lame "what is gluten?" talk is over. Is it time to pop the champagne yet?

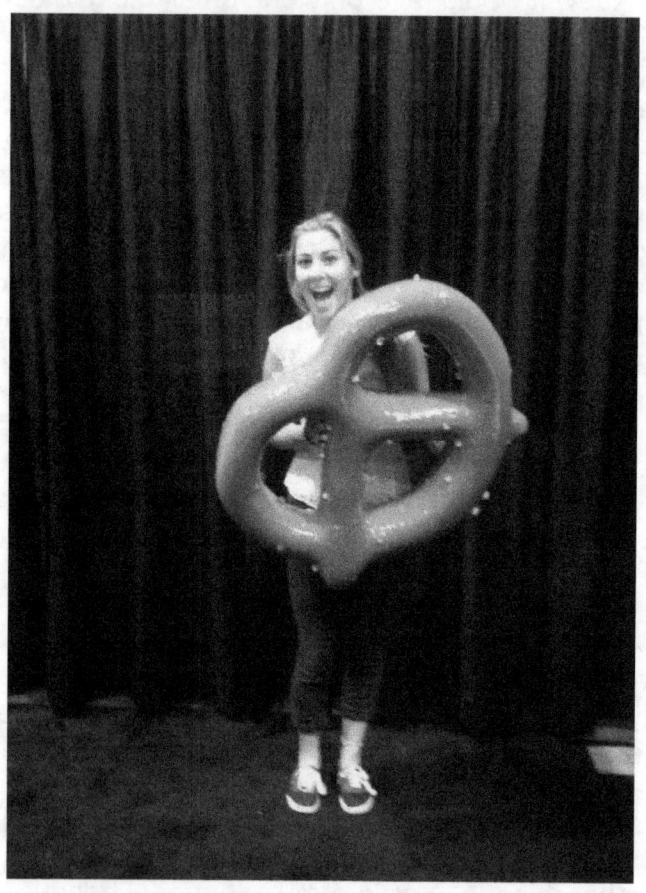

Now on to **BIGGER**, better, tastier, *and* MORE EXCITING THINGS!

# THE GRITTY AND ENTERTAINING PARTS

**People really do make things so much more difficult!**

# LET'S TALK ABOUT WHAT HAPPENS WHEN YOU TELL PEOPLE YOU ARE GLUTEN FREE

This is seriously one of the most exciting topics for me believe it or not. I won't lie to you and say that I enjoy telling people that I am gluten free because that is just absurd and I have dealt with so much 'smack' that people talk that I almost don't even want to bring it up. I am what I'd like to call a "risk taker" or "adrenaline junkie". These statements would mean that when I go out to eat, instead of asking the server is this Gluten free? I just speculate and order what I want anyways. My mom (sadly) sometimes still does it for me because I would rather risk it than to admit I have special dietary needs. I also do not really know how to reply to people most of the time when they ask me why I am gluten free. So, here is a nice little list of some of the craziest things I have heard so far about my "choosing to be GF".
(I am also very curious to hear what all you have heard so far!)

- **Me: "Ma'am is the grilled, swiss, barbecue chicken gluten free?"**
**Waitress: Well it has swiss cheese on it so..."**
**Me: "Never mind can I please have the grilled chicken without a bun and a side of fruit?"**
I was actually floored that the poor gal thought swiss cheese was gluten. But, I guess I was in her shoes at one point also. If she genuinely did not know what gluten was, I can not hold anything against her! Also, this was one of my 'risk taker' moments.

- **"Hey, I tried this new recipe the other day... Oh... That's right... You can't eat it anyways!"**
GIMME THE RECIPE!!!!
I will FIND a new way to cook it!

- **"You're just exaggerating Andrea. It can't be that bad can it?"**
I appreciate your genuine concern you total jerk. But yes, it's really that bad! Sometimes it's worse! Actually, it's always worse than what I tell you... When I say "no thank you" you should think back to your preschool days... Hasn't anyone ever taught you that no means no? I was respectfully declining the death trap you were trying to hand me. But when you ask questions such as these, and you ask them in a facetious manner, I feel belittled and I may not respond back in a very calm way. Actually, when I'm asked questions about if I'm exaggerating, I feel my face turn red, I start to sweat, and I feel my blood pressure rise. Not to mention the blood vessels in my eyes I feel popping as I'm trying to hold my breath and bite my tongue. So, don't ever ask me this! Mmk? Thanks!

- **"So, what can you eat?"**
Surprisingly enough, I can eat a lot! And I try to focus on the fact that I can eat tacos! I can eat mostly any fruit, vegetable, meat and cheese (even though I try to avoid it). (**Warning:** I choose to stay away from dairy because I'm lactose intolerant and it goes hand in hand with gluten intolerance. Please do not mistake that as me disliking cheese!) I always like focusing on the whole foods but there are lots of new gluten free items making their way to the mainstream market! There are some awesome products and restaurants that offer GF options and I must say that I've had some awesome experiences, as well as some terrible ones but the awesome ones generally outweigh the few bad experiences I've had.

## • "So you mean to tell me, that means that you can't eat..."

For the most part, when this comes up in a topic, the answer is NO I can NOT eat that. Thanks for shoving my nose in it! My dad is actually notorious for bringing things home that I can not eat. I used to be upset about it, anymore though, I will make something equally delicious and tell him he is not allowed to have any!

## • "You can still eat the fried chicken if you pull the breading off the outside!"

NO! Thanks for the after thought though you jerk face. All that I would be doing if I ate that darn chicken would be saying "hey gluten monster wanna have a toilet date and maybe netflix and chill for a week?" Thanks but no thanks. I would rather eat the canned green beans that you laid out on the table to make it a more colorful and healthier dinner! I will just sit here and smell the greasy goodness that is dripping through your fingers instead.

## • "Oh you are so skinny why are you Gluten Free?"

Actually yes I am skinny, but no I did not choose the GF life to lose weight. The reality of this was that I had lost so much weight before going gluten free that I actually looked sickly. Since having gone gluten free I have gained weight back because my body is finally starting to digest food and absorb nutrients!

## • "You eat gluten free... Your new nickname is Gluten Freak."

Thanks Kid. This is honestly a super exciting one I have heard from my brother. Thanks you little brat. I could not even be mad at him because he chose this one when I was sick one day and he was bringing me something to eat. Poor kid won't admit he loves me but he does usually go out of his way to do awesome things for me.

# • "Maybe you will grow out of it."

No, I won't grow out of it! My insides could take up to two or three years to heal and even then, I have no desire to eat gluten again!

# • "Oh you're one of 'those' gluten free people."

Actually I just want everyone to understand that, every time I hear this specific statement, a very violent nature in me comes out and I have to say several prayers that I do not kick you in the shin. I hope I am not the only one who feels this way. I am not sure why I get so defensive over this specific statement, but it sure does stick like a knife, and at that point I have to go into detail as to why I chose gluten free. I usually go ahead and tell them the very easy to explain, "it makes me sick, makes me have very intimate relations with the bathroom, and I get to go meet new doctors and nurses and pay very high hospital bills when I eat things that look and taste so darn good. So no, I am not one of 'those' people. I would also like it if you did not refer to me as such." Oh and by the way, I wish you would have known me before I had stomach issues, I would probably beat you in a pie eating or taco eating contest (I actually may still beat you in a taco eating contest, but I haven't opened up about my taco addiction yet!)

# • "Since you are gluten free, you must eat so much healthier!"

Actually yes I do, but not because of the GF products. The reality of this statement is actually a grueling truth. Processed gluten free items and mixes have so much more sugar, sodium, and additives in them because there is really no other way to make the mixture taste palatable without gluten. I AM relatively healthy because I stay away from processed foods as much as I can, and I enjoy eating whole foods more than any of the processed foods. (I still like my cookies, cupcakes and taco shells!)

· **"I hope what you have isn't contagious."**
Ha, you can not be serious, can you? Listen, you can NOT get the gluten problems that I have from breathing the same air, touching something I have touched, or kissing me. It just simply isn't possible. UNLESS your body is as hateful towards you as mine is towards me and decides to just randomly start rejecting food that you absolutely love and would not mind having a plethora of, hidden under your bed or maybe owning stock in. (Also, yes I have a stash of my gluten free snacks hidden. Mom and Dad... Do not get any ideas!)

# ALLOW ME TO CLEAR UP SOME MISCONCEPTIONS ABOUT BEING GF

I have written about some of the things I have heard but I want to address a few issues I have run across. I want to make sure that everyone understands what being gluten free entails as well as some of the misunderstandings that have been presumed.

- **I am not jumping on the 'bandwagon.' This is actually a necessity for my health. I am not eating gluten free for fun.**
- **I never want anyone to take it personally when I deny food from them. Even if it is made specifically for me and is gluten free.**

I love the gesture and it means the world to me. However, sometimes I am not willing to take the chance. Not because I do not trust you, but there is a chance that your utensils, pots and pans, and ingredients could all be holding those gluten monster particles.

- **Gluten Intolerance is not the same as a food allergy!**

It affects my whole body and sometimes does not cause a reaction immediately after ingesting the gluten. Sometimes it takes a few days but that does not mean that it does not hurt me!

- **I sometimes feel left out and sad when everyone is enjoying nice treats, and I am eating a frozen pre-made pizza.**

## • I can not control how I feel and I never know when a flare up is going to happen.

This could mean that I am going to bail on lots of events and I will hate every minute of it. I have no idea how my body will react to what I ate three days ago. So please be patient with me.

## • No, there is not a magic pill to make it go away.

There is lots of research being done to find a cure or even a remedy but, nothing definitive yet.

## • One small teaspoon of flour will hurt me!

No matter how much gluten is in something, it will make me sick. Even if your wooden spoon was used to make brownies a week ago and you used it to stir my gluten free pasta. It could contaminate my pasta and leave me enjoying the company of a good book and a fancy commode.

## • Gluten Free food isn't nearly as bad as you think it is.

## • Before we eat, or even order food, please point me to the nearest restroom. I like to always know where it is!

## • Please don't tell me it is safe for me to eat if you don't know.

It is the same as feeding me food that has poison in it. The only difference is that it takes much longer to heal from.

## • I hate explaining my problems to you.

If I am taking my time explaining what gluten intolerance is to you, please pay attention and don't act judgemental. I don't want to waste my time or yours and I surely do not enjoy complaining about my 'bad stomach' to anyone, much less someone who shows no interest.

## • If you eat pasta with your fork, don't try to eat off of my plate with the gluten covered fork!

You can be cross contaminating my currently safe food with your little gluten monster demon fork.

## • I read every label on every box and bag that i pick up at the supermarket.

I really do not enjoy doing this. I feel obsessive! But, I also don't enjoy feeling sick.

## • I get tired of eating salads!

Sure, they are amazing, and they taste great! But, not every day, two or three meals a day.

## • I feel like a kid in a candy store when a restaurant has a gluten free menu!

## • When I am hurting or sick, I will still smile and do my best to make it seem like I am okay.

# CONVENIENCE AND BEING GF

Do not get your hopes up because there isn't any convenience in eating gluten free. Not that convenience is completely obsolete for the GF family! It is however much more risky and difficult to achieve and also requires a bit of work. And let's be completely honest with ourselves here, when that silly 'work' word is thrown around, can you really call it convenience?

So, have you started this gluten free lifestyle yet? It sounds glamorous doesn't it? Well it really is (or can be at least)! I use the fact that I am gluten free to my advantage and I embrace it more than most people are comfortable with. Have you ever used the "sorry I can't eat that because I don't know if it is safe?" I have! I turned down hamburgers, cooked in gravy, that came out of a can. I was more than obliged to use the fact that I am GF to my advantage!

So, instead of sitting over there sulking and hugging your M&M's and salad because those are your 'safe' foods, jump up off the couch, pause Netflix, and start using Pinterest! They have tons of food ideas, jokes, and not to mention product ideas! I will give you some time to sit and be sad over the fact that a deep fried cookie may not be in your future but, think of the positives! You will find foods that actually taste better than the original! And, your cooking style may actually be a bit healthier and oh man, there are so many other reasons to look at the bright side!

Keep your chin up my dear, the sunshine is only a few minutes away. (Especially in Florida where the sideways down pouring of rain only lasts about 10 minutes!)

# DO YOU EVER MISS...?

HECK YES! Sometimes I miss eating "normal food", but other days I couldn't tell the difference between "normal" and GF options. I really do however, miss eating convenient (or quick grab) foods, and greasy foods and quite frankly, I miss being able to eat whatever the heck I feel like eating! Actually, in the beginning stages of learning about what gluten free really entailed, I drove past the Florida Fair and I cried, because I came to a realization that I could never eat funnel cake, fried strawberries, fried Oreos or a deep crust pizza again!

I have found some awesome substitutes but none as good as that deep fried, crunchy and greasy goodness. I have surely done my fair share of trying gluten free items and exploring new things! That being said, there are tons of items that I guarantee you will try and hate. Between that gritty texture, gross after taste, greasy coating left in your mouth, or the funky smells that protrude from the oven when you are brave enough to actually give some of these products a try, it sounds like a lose, lose situation. But, there are a few that are just absolutely delicious and some are not as costly as you may think! Actually, I have found some substitutes that are just fantastic and I think that some of them are actually better than the gluten filled versions. I am not as skilled in the 'make my own almond milk and almond flour' category even though I really do wish I could because that would save me so much money! So, for those of you who are lazy, not skilled in the kitchen, or looking for a quick replacement, allow me to be of assistance by sharing some of the foods I actually have come to love!

# MY GLORIOUS LIST
# OF STAPLE FOODS

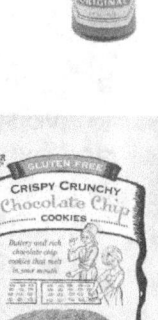

- **Daiya GF and Dairy Free Cheesecake- Publix Frozen** (It is actually fantastic!)
- **Trader Joe's GF Chocolate Chip Cookies**
- **Kind Bars**
- **Udi's GF Macaroni and Cheese**
- **Udi's GF Blueberry Muffins**
- **Betty Crocker GF Devil's Food Cake Mix** (Probably the best cake mix I have found! Will also probably be at least one layer of my wedding cake one day)
- **Wine**
- **Toufayan Bakeries Gluten Free Wraps** (I enjoy the spinach)
- **Chocolate Chex Mix**
- **Lance's GF Cheddar Cheese Sandwich Crackers** (Comparable to Ritz crackers but less cheesy and greasy)
- **San-J Tamari GF Soy Sauce**
- **Rice noodles and GF branded noodles**
- **Corn tortilla shells** (I turn tacos into a daily thing! Just wait until I get into my taco addiction... It's coming!)
- **Wine!**
- **Fresh Fruit and Veggies** (I ALWAYS have apples, spinach, lettuce, cabbage, cucumber, carrot, tomato, red and sweet onion, potatoes and sweet potatoes.)
- **Dole Mixed Fruit Cups with 100% Juice**
- **Cholula Hot Sauce** (I put this stuff on EVERYTHING!)
- **Fresh Eggs**

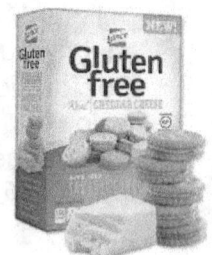

- **Frozen Fruit and some Veggies**
(Used in smoothies, meals or random other happenings in the kitchen)
- **Wine!!**
- **Tortilla chips**
(Make sure they are only corn and actually say gluten free!)
- **Udi's Hot Dog Buns**
- **Live G Free Stuffed Sandwiches**
 (Similar to a Hot Pocket)
- **Ian's Breaded Chicken Nuggets**
- **Publix GF Blueberry Waffles**
(Trust me when I say, these are the best darn waffles ever!)
- **Applesauce**
- **Udi's GF Pizza**
(I actually don't eat this that much anymore since avoiding processed foods. It is however, excellent when it is cooked a little longer than it says to cook it. The more cooked it is, the crispier it is. I think that is the best way I have ever enjoyed eating it! Sad thing is, I had to find that out by burning mine so much that it was almost completely charred, but even though it was burnt it was one of the best GF pizza cooking sessions I have had!)
- **Oh and since we were on the topic of things I enjoy keeping stocked... WINE!!!**

Many of these items are the more convenient things that we get lucky enough to be able to enjoy. They are gluten free either by the processing they do or by natural occurrence. However, these are things that I tend to have stocked in my cabinets, freezer and refrigerator at any given point in time!
Now it's your turn to get off the couch (when you start feeling better) jump in your car (or walk if you are feeling ambitious) and go explore your local supermarket! See what all they have to offer you may be surprised. (Places I go shopping are listed in the resources.)

# RELATIONSHIPS AND GF?
# HA! IF ONLY!

It is no surprise that when you choose the Gluten Free Lifestyle, or in my case, the GF Lifestyle chose you, that your relationships all change. For a while I was nearly a basket case any time someone had asked me to go out to eat with them. I would immediately feel signs of anxiety as well as stress, wondering if I should eat before I went out or if I should just eat a salad, and sometimes even that would make me feel sick.

# Friends/Acquaintances/jerks

One perk of this lifestyle change is that when you start taking care of yourself and focusing on making yourself better, you attract better people and you somehow in an almost magical way, see all of the people who are bad for you go POOF into a magic cloud of 'jerk dust'. (Notice the lowercase J in jerks for the title!)

I stopped going out and drinking and partying and eating out multiple times a week. I started to go to bed earlier, pray more (for strength and for support), I spent more time with family and there you have it! I was down to less than a handful of friends.

For those jerks that decided that I was too much of a hassle for them, I appreciate the way you made me feel worse than I already did. However, to the loving, caring, patient friends that stuck around and helped me do research for gluten free restaurants and meals. You are truly angels. You helped me when I was sick and on the bathroom floor. You helped me not to goof and buy something that would make me feel sick. And you stuck around for the movie days I had to have, even when we had big plans for adventure that I had to bail on because I was too sick to get out of the house or dorm.

# Family (you gotta love 'em)

When it comes to family, my parents did not quite believe that it was a gluten problem either. They were standing right where I was only a few months ago (until I went and tried out that lovely "Whole 30" I talked about). They thought I was jumping on the band-wagon or that I had lost my mind. I could not convince anyone to believe what I had to say about the way different foods were affecting the way I felt. I learned quickly that Gluten was a huge problem and contributor to my health problems. They were looking in all other areas of health for answers. Was my thyroid off balance? How about my sleeping patterns? Maybe I am just stressed or anxious? Maybe I had an eating disorder? All of these things had been discussed in one form or another and it was exhausting honestly. Because, at the end of the day I knew, whatever I was eating and putting into my body is what was causing me the most problems. I came home from vacation and decided on that day, that I was not going back to eating Gluten and I haven't! This has not been an easy road to have traveled on but it seems to be getting easier with each passing day.

I started to notice that I was pulling away from my family in the way that communication really ceased because they never really seemed to listen to what I had to say about my health and they would assume their own theories. It took me a few months before I was able to get back up on my feet and my mother noticed a big change in me... I had not been sick in nearly a full month! No doctor visits, no seriously bad gluten attacks and I was feeling great, gaining some weight and I started to look happy again! This was the turning point, where I started to have some more support.

After being gluten free for nearly 6 months my family as a whole decided to see what I was ranting and raving about with the "Whole 30" diet. They gave it a shot, and they have also had some excellent results! My father has lost a ton of weight and is now more aware of how he feels after eating certain foods and my mom is also doing great in her health journey! As for my brother, he still enjoys fast food and candy but he will come around.

# Going to Parties and being social and such

Going to events has changed dramatically since going GF. Every few months at church we have a 'dinner on the grounds' which is basically a potluck. Potluck in gluten free lingo = NIGHTMARE, you better plan on starving, and forget the food, focus on socializing and work on becoming a more social person you couch potato!

Even though I may be gluten free, I often time engage in what I like to call 'risky behavior'. This means that I hop up and go make myself a plate of food even though I know that I could pay for it later on. I almost always decide that it is a price I am willing to pay and as if by some miracle, I have not yet been glutened at a church function! Hallelujah! Oh, before I get off of talking about going to church… Once in awhile we also have a communion at church. For those of you who are not aware of what that is, it is a gathering of the church body and there are communion crackers and grape juice or wine. At the Last Supper in the Bible, Jesus says to do this in memory of him. We break the bread (communion crackers in remembrance of the body of Christ) and we drink the wine (in remembrance of the blood of Christ). This is a sacred and meaningful practice however, I can not eat the communion crackers! The last time we did this, I picked out a cracker when the tray was passed around because I felt disrespectful if I didn't. I held onto the cracker until the prayer was over and I handed it to my mom (she's a trooper) to eat and I think it was the funniest look that she has ever had on her face when she looked down to take it from me. Naturally, I grabbed the biggest piece in the basket! And, now she had to eat it without choking to death! (The communion crackers are matzah so, dry and unleavened and hard to eat without liquid.) Moving on.

I have also gone to two other events in the past six months that were hosted by close friends of mine. One event was a wedding and the other was a graduation party. At both events, there was a specially marked gluten free dessert! There were other options for dinner as well but the most exciting part was that they had purchased a separate GF dessert, all because I had been so vocal over time about my health concerns and my decision to eat gluten free! This was an amazing change in pace and it opened my eyes that maybe my world was not going to end after all. I was thanking God for sending friends my way that care so much! It makes it so much easier when support is there.

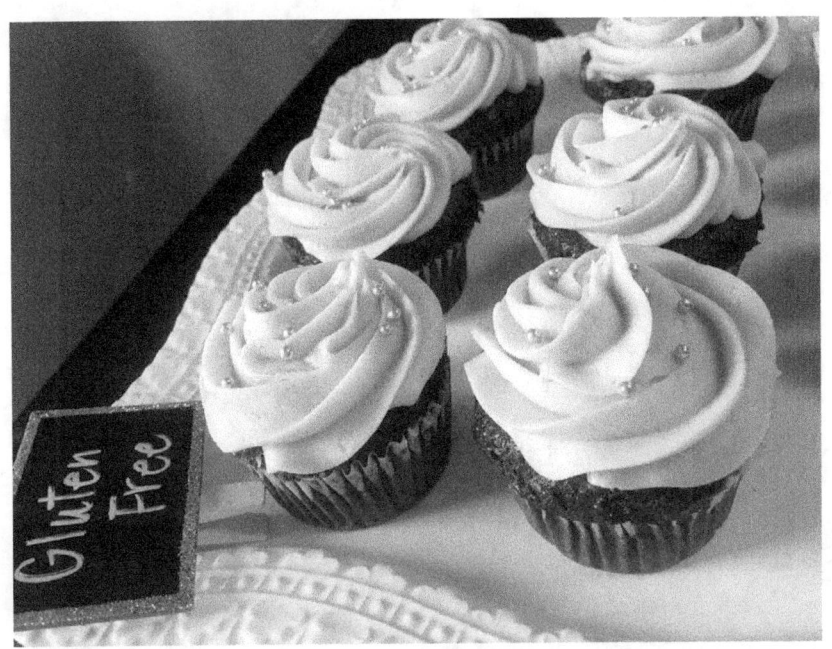

I have had people from all over the place asking me about how I went GF and for my advice on diets and on the "Whole 30". I can not give much advice aside from this...

You **ABSOLUTELY** have to want change
In Order for change to happen

# WHAT HAPPENS WHEN I AM ATTACKED BY THE NASTY GLUTEN MONSTER?

# HERE COMES THE... UH OH!

## Yes, there is an entire chapter for this!

Let's be completely honest here. It is never pretty when I have been glutened and I have a long list of references for people who can attest to that! There are some days when I have stomach cramps, slight nausea, and dizziness and it goes away if I force myself to work through it. There are other days when I am standing at work and I am slurring my words, can't focus, and am struggling to walk straight or function at all! Those days are frustrating and generally have everyone concerned because my hand-eye coordination drops to the level of a town drunk. If you think that is funny I am glad I can make you laugh! I may be frustrated about it but it always livens up the work place when the jokes start to turn to the "Andrea where is your brain today?" My response to comments like those usually take a few moments, especially on long, brain fog days such as those; but they end up along the lines of well my brain has gone down the toilet drain, just like the gluten filled whatever I ate.

I have been glutened quite a few times and let me just say, if you are new to the gluten intolerance I want to go ahead and say I am sympathizing with you; but, I refuse to sulk with you. I refuse to sulk over the gluten monster attacks that I have because it may seem miserable at the time, but my goodness looking back at some of the insane things that happen are quite comedic. I am very shy to tell people outside of my very VERY close knit circle some of the things that have happened when I mess up and get glutened. I however, have decided that if I am going through it, someone else probably is as well. You may be scared to death by some of the things that you see (I still wonder if some of the things that happen are normal or paranormal, they are so weird) and I do not blame you one bit, but I want you to know that you are not alone!

There are millions of us that are suffering from food allergies, gluten intolerance, Celiac Disease, and many other diseases or allergies or health problems. Why are we not talking about this stuff? Why is the fact that we are struggling with not pooping our pants after someone lies and says "sure it is safe for you to eat" being hidden from everyone? Well, I think it is time to shed some light on the details of what each of us goes through and maybe you can relate to it, or maybe you know someone who is going through it, and now you can understand all of those nitty gritty details that they are sparing you. You may want to think twice before reading this chapter if you want to continue seeing us all as royalty and as people who are perfectly normal, because we aren't and I am about to start showing you what we really go through!

Photo: Our Thanksgiving dinner! This was our first family holiday gathering eating completely gluten free! GF gravy, roasted turkey, green bean casserole, and so much more! Oh did I forget to mention Moscato for
desert?

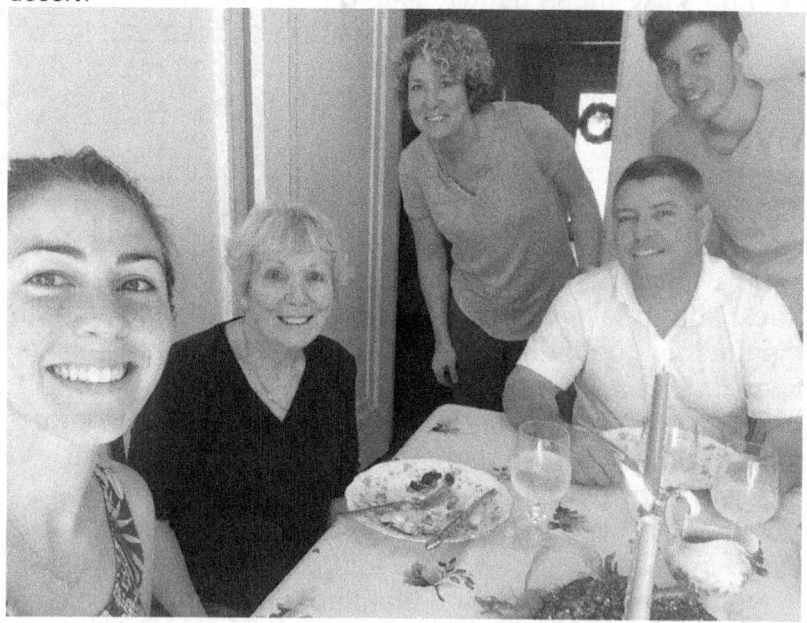

Since you've read this far into the book you might as well keep reading! This is where all of the stories and truths come out, some that you may be able to relate to, and some you may just enjoy snickering at (because laughing may cause you to poop your pants), besides, laughter (or in my case snickering) is the best medicine anyways. Either way, if you're sitting on the toilet reading this right now because you have been attacked by the gluten monster, you should feel like you have company and not feel so bad, because I wrote half of this book while I was on the porcelain throne. Yup, it's true! I gluten poisoned myself and I spent about 3 days on a toilet. As a matter of a fact, I am finally starting to be able to eat food again two weeks later, and even be more than a mile away from the good ole ladies room where I've been making the magic for this lovely book happen!

You may be wondering why I am so positive and why I am okay with the situation at hand. Well, that's actually an easy one! I won't lead you on to believe that every day is a good day because it really isn't. I never know from one day to the next how I will feel. I take each day as it is handed to me! This means that on my good days, I embrace them and act as if nothing could possibly bring me down. And on my bad days, I use it as my way to catch up on my Netflix shows and movies, and dream about the food I get to make when I can stand up straight again!

I do my best not to sulk and feel sorry for myself because, I know people who have it far worse than I do. Instead, I try to focus on how to make myself healthier, happier, and a better person!

# DO NOT MESS WITH MY FOOD!

# SHARING FOOD

## WHAT'S THAT GOT TO DO WITH THE PRICE...

Speaking of eating food! I am pretty picky about sharing my food and who I share it with. My boyfriend, my brother, and my parents are NOTORIOUS for stealing my food and it drives me absolutely insane. If you're at all aware of how painful going to the grocery store is to shop for gluten free food, you understand that the items are much more expensive (my wallet is empty) and it's usually an optical illusion to make it look like you received the same amount of product as you would normally purchase. Stop! It's a trap! It's all a lie and it's terrible. I went to the supermarket and purchased a bag of cookies that we're actually pretty decently sized, or so I thought! I was dumbfounded to see that the inside had two hard plastic separators to divide the cookies into two sections, and then they were plastic wrapped to keep it fresh inside of a plastic bag! So, what the heck did I pay for here? The plastic they kept wasting in order to fool me into thinking that I was getting more? Or was I paying for the amazing cookie that was small enough to feed a sugar ant? I have learned that the packaging for gluten free products is not the way to judge how much you're actually receiving. You should always expect that you're paying for one third of the size of the portion and maybe even half of the size of a normal gluten filled product.

All of that being said, I don't like to share my very expensive treats when I finally splurge on them. I have my own cabinet in the kitchen, filled with all of the random gluten free gems that I don't want to share with anyone else. I even try to play the "it's gluten free, you wouldn't like it" card, so that nobody wants to eat those scrumptious cookies and cupcakes I'm stashing. But, in the case of my family, they don't care if it's gross or not! If it's sweet and it's there, they will devour it! As for the boyfriend, I think he is the same exact way, he won't ever admit it! He uses the excuse, "well if you're eating it, I want to try it and maybe we can both just eat gluten free." Um, NO! Can you please eat your name brand chocolate chip, two dollars a box cookies, so I can enjoy the five cookies I got in a false advertising plastic bag for eight dollars?

# EATING SHOULDN'T BE A CRIME

I am guilty of eating at least 5 meals a day. I have some very odd tendencies due to that fact. For instance, I mentioned that I have my own cabinet in the kitchen, but I also have snacks in my purse, my room, my car, and anywhere else I can stash them for the pure sake of, I am hungry and need something to eat! But, it is more than that! I actually try to have food stashed away just in case I am out and about and nobody has anything that I can eat. I want to have those safe snacks with me. I guarantee you that not everywhere you go is going to have a safe gluten free option and that is where the crazy comes in.

So, with all of that being said, I am one of those people who goes to a party whether it be a birthday party, Fourth of July party, or whatever random event it may be, and I take a bag of snacks. I always offer to bring something out of pure common courtesy (and sometimes a little bit of concern for the explosion of my insides) but when they say "just bring yourself and a smile", I bring myself, a bag of snacks, and a glass full of wine! Depending on the event I choose my glass of wine wisely it is either half a bottle or a glass that fits the full bottle. In which case, I may just carry the bottle into the party! When it comes time to eat, I assure the host of the party that I've already eaten and I go outside to my car to "check on something" or "make a phone call" and I stuff my face with whatever quick goodies I have stuffed away at that point in time. Sometimes I have a full meal sitting in the cooler and I eat it as quick as I can before anyone gets suspicious!

So, yes I still go to gatherings, and yes I still eat at them! But, no I do not always act "normal" at said gatherings. Oh and for some of you who have birthday cake at your gatherings… You should know that you all suck, and I go home after leaving your party and make cupcakes that I can actually eat because they look so darn good! (And, now I am craving a nice delicious triple iced cupcake.)

Photo: This is a nice little collection of some of the goodies I can be caught carrying at any given point in time. I will say this though, if you see me around town, don't you dare try to stop me and ask me for my granola bars because those are like gold to me!

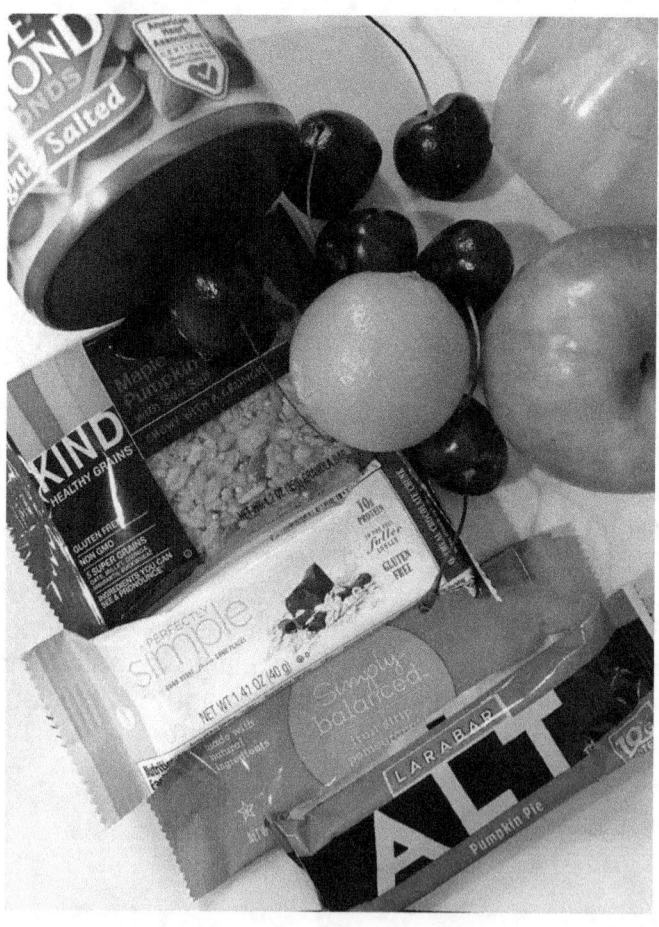

# WHAT HAPPENS WHEN YOU ARE SICK?

Listen, there is absolutely no right answer to this question! Learning how to handle an upset tummy without the normal crackers and sprite is a huge learning curve for me. We have all grown up with those "comfort foods" when we are sick and I noticed that all of mine have been taken away! I have switched over to eating apples, rice, oranges, Alkaseltzer (this is a major food group in my life), salads, apple sauce, and potatoes. Oh and on those I need a sweet treat or something to fill my belly days I find that good ole chocolate Chex cereal mix!
find that good ole chocolate chex cereal mix!

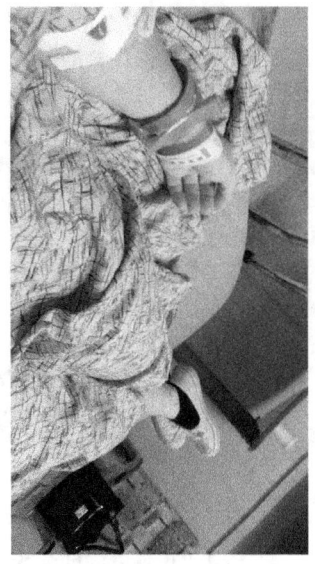

Photo: This was one of my many hospital trips as you can tell by that lovely, flowy, and quite risky dress that they provided! I was definitely on a soup diet for this trip and was craving anything solid to eat since I had not eaten anything solid in days! I was excited to enjoy some nice cheddar broccoli soup also when I got out of the hospital. (Because naturally as a gluten free, lactose intolerant gal, I wanted the soup that tends to have it all!) And yes, I have socks with my shoes on! Don't judge me! This was one of those times where I was not able to dress myself! I enjoy looking at these photos!

# BEING GLUTENED
# TO THE MAX

   I complain, I complain a lot when I have been glutened! Actually, I start complaining the minute it happens because I know that it will start feeling uncomfortable in a few minutes, and it will escalate to me wanting to go die in a deep dark hole in a few days. I have had a few rather funny gluten poisoning stories but this last time is one of my favorites. I say it is one of my favorites because I did it to myself and I knew it only moments after it happened. You know how I mentioned that you need to read every label on every piece of food you buy in the store? YOU DO! Because I went shopping and decided that (against my better judgement) I wanted to splurge and buy a nice little thing of ice cream! I went to the section that was on sale and started looking through all of the awesome flavors that they had. I grabbed one, skimmed the back and didn't see any major ingredient no, no's (such as cookies, caramels, wheat and such) that stood out as something I could not have. So, I threw it in the basket and walked to check out. I got back to the house and took a bite of the ice cream eager to taste the coffee and caramel flavor (oops, didn't I say caramel was dangerous) and it was absolutely delicious! As I was scooping the second bite out of the container I was reading the ingredients and I felt a knot in my stomach as I continued to read "Dry Malt Extract (Barley)". WHO PUTS BARLEY IN ICE CREAM! And, WHY DIDN'T I SEE THAT!? I had already shoved the second spoonful into my mouth and I ran to the bathroom to spit it out and rinse my mouth out. (As if I had not already invited the gluten monster into my gut!)

   I started to feel stomach cramps about 5 minutes after eating that small bite I had taken when I first got home and I knew that the rest of the week was going to be a roller coaster, and trust me, it has been!

The next night was a night where I made some amazing fish tacos! I mean, they were fantastic and I was so proud of them! The entire yard smelled like a taqueria and I was more proud of this than any of my other cooking achievements. I could eat tacos every single day of the week, possibly multiple times a day, and I would be satisfied! If you're making dinner, throw it in a taco shell you may be surprised! (I will share some of my taco ideas later on, no worries!) But anyways, I was okay after eating but just started to feel a little grumbly in my tummy.

The next night, I cooked cajun stir fry sausage, beans, rice and peppers and it was amazing! It was super spicy however and I thought that maybe I made it too spicy to handle. I was tired all day but never really felt like I was going to have a gluten attack until about 9:00 that night. All of a sudden I was sweating, shivering because I was cold, my stomach sounded like a herd of elephants, and I started to feel pressure in my stomach that made me think that I was a gas canister sitting out in the sun ready to explode! I hung in there thinking that it would pass, maybe it was just gas or maybe I just was too tired. I could not be any more wrong! I was running to the bathroom and had my pants unzipped and to my knees before I even got there. The gluten monster has struck again! I was up until 2:30 in the morning running back and forth from my couch and my toilet while writing this lovely book.

The next day was the same thing. I sat on the couch all day writing because I was too scared to leave the house! I did however, force myself to get up and do some yard work but only small amounts of yard work at a time because I was completely exhausted and was feeling way worse than I remember. (Every single time I get glutened, it always seems worse than the last episode. Generally it is because I can not remember the last gluten attack, they all run together anymore!)

After I was done pooping every three or four hours for two days, I finally started to gain a little more strength! I was able to get up and move around! I felt dizzy, weak, and nauseous but let me tell you how much I ate that day. I ate like a champ! I ate anything and everything in sight because I was sucking down apple sauce and eating oranges the day before. It was time to regain some energy and strength. I was still exhausted feeling and would continue to feel that way for at least another few days but man I must say getting off that darn couch was the best thing I could ever imagine! I am not the type of person who enjoys sitting down for more than an hour at a time. I like to wear myself out and work as hard as I can during the day, so that when it turns dark outside, I can crawl into bed and go to sleep without a problem! Sitting inside sick for two days, makes me feel like the world is coming to an end! (Unless I have a project such as this to keep me busy and occupied!) This was a fairly short gluten attack (I was in pain for only a few days, but could still feel the effects of it two weeks later.) from that measling taste of heavenly, coffee caramel goodness! I am always super excited when the gluten problems last a week or less! That means that I can sit for a day or two or sometimes the full month and then I will be okay!

# ALWAYS SICK
# BEFORE VACATION

It never fails that right before vacation, I am always sick! For some reason or another I can avoid sickness all the way up until I am getting packed and ready to jump on the road. I was headed to the Florida Keys on vacation this time, and this has been planned for nearly a year! About two months before vacation I was feeling horrible. I was contributing it to stress or to being exhausted and working way too hard and running my body into the ground, but I still couldn't tell you exactly what was happening. I know that I was exhausted all the time, did not want to eat anything so I would have to force myself to eat, and I was sleeping almost 10 hours every night! Now, as an understanding of what I was doing for work, I was helping with some demolition and construction in a rental home, working a few nights as a waitress, and doing all of the yard work around the house. I was exhausted and the awesome 90 + degree weather in Florida did not make it any easier!

I started to wonder if I was struggling with a relapse of Mono (I had mono when I was in high school). I was cranky, miserable, never smiled anymore because I did not have the energy to do so, and I was really miserable with myself so I can not imagine how anyone put up with me during these few months.

I started to take Dessicated Adrenal to boost energy levels as well as chewable probiotics to start getting my gut health back to where it needed to be! Exciting enough to say, I was smiling again and enjoyed being around people more! It took time but I came out on top!

Photo: This is what my fishing trips tend to look like! Lot's of wine to drink and dozens of fish to clean!

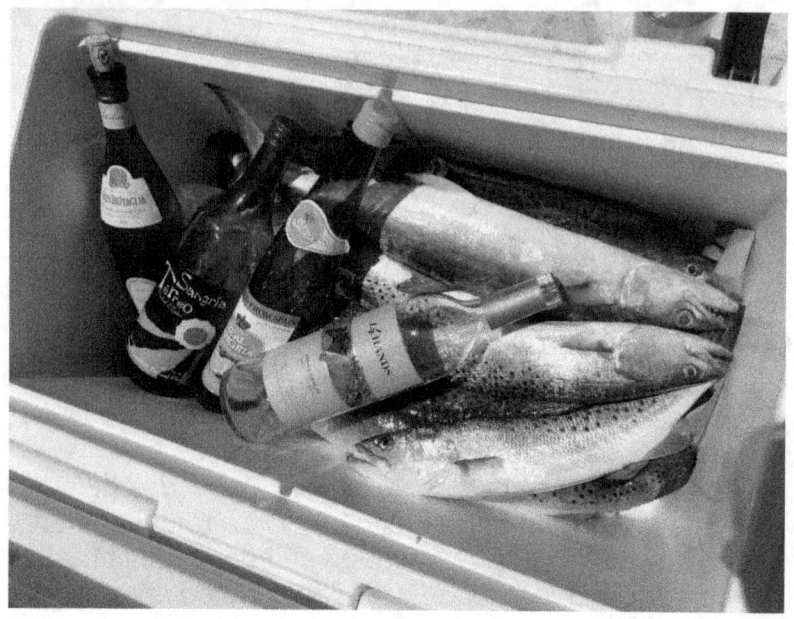

# WHAT DOES YOUR MEDICINE CABINET LOOK LIKE?

To be honest, I am completely blessed not to have a ton of medicines that I am required to take. I do however, have quite the arsenal of meds for those random happenings when medicine might help. So, here goes a list of meds that I always have stashed away!

- **Ibuprofen-** Great for any aches or pains that may happen since I get headaches and sometimes I am clumsy (I walk into walls, tables, and trip over random items, leading to copious amounts of pain!) This is a staple that I carry in my purse at any given point in time!
- **Loratadine-** Allergy meds. Need I say more?
- **Benadryl-** Because, sometimes I need a more powerful and quick acting allergy medicine. In the cases of my random need to snuggle with cats and my eyes swelling shut!
- **Soverign Silver-** A great way to build your immune system. (I added a link in the references section for this product)
- **Vitamin D3-** Also used to build my immune system and help get over any amount of sickness I may have.
- **Gas and Heartburn Relief-** It helps with EVERYTHING!
- **Dessicated Adrenal-** Helps boost energy levels when I have been glutened.
- **Lactose Chewables-** I always have it with me. But honestly, do I ever use it? No.
- **Calcium Vitamins**
- **Multi-Vitamins**
- **Chewable Probiotics**

And the list goes on! However, these are the most used medicines in my cabinet and they are how I get through daily life whether it be the vitamins, allergies, or what not's. Just remember to **double check any medicine or vitamins you may take!** Sometimes they hide gluten into these "helpful" items! Find what works for you and maximize your health.

# BE SURE TO CONSULT WITH YOUR DOCTOR BEFORE TRYING ANY NEW MEDICINE!

# ALCOHOL!!!

Let's be honest, this is one of the more exciting parts of the book. Therefore, I dedicated a chapter solely to it! Please understand that I am not an alcoholic! I also do not promote drinking alcohol because, it really isn't good for you in any way shape or form and I don't care how many different published articles there are that say otherwise.

All of that being said, I enjoy my occasional drink and I am quite the wine fanatic!

Before I realized I had any stomach or gut issues I was a major whiskey, scotch, and beer snob! I enjoyed drinking my whiskey and scotch straight and I loved my craft beers cold! All of that changed though, when I started researching what living gluten free entailed. I came to the sad (and wrong) realization that I would never be able to enjoy any of these drinks again! I thought that drinking anything made from wheat, barley, rye, or anything else for that matter would cause me major problems.

Are you ready to hear the most exciting part?
## I WAS WRONG!

# YOU CAN DRINK ALL OF THE FOLLOWING

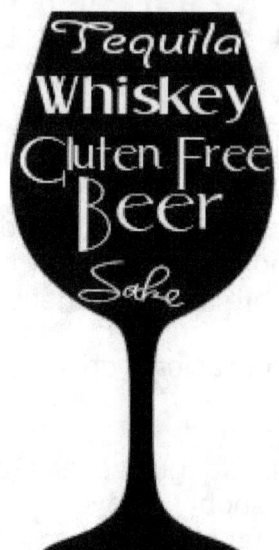 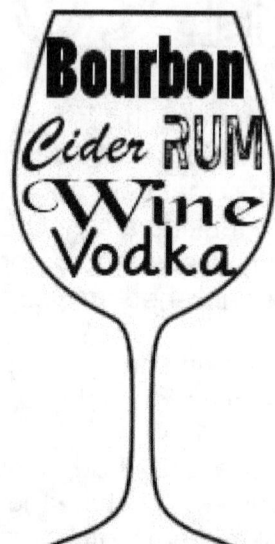

Gluten Free Beer

Cider

Vodka

Rum

Tequila

Whiskey

Bourbon

Wine

Sake

# BUT WAIT... THERE'S MORE YOU NEED TO KNOW!

No matter what you choose to drink, be safe and remember to **read the labels. <u>NOT ALL</u> alcohol is made the same!** Some Celiacs are able to drink certain whiskey and bourbon without any problem due to the distilling process, others are not so lucky. Make sure that you do a little more research before you decide that you want to go crazy!

To be safe with drinking vodka you may want to make sure that you are drinking potato vodka and **BEWARE OF FLAVORED VODKA!**

Wine is generally more of a safe drink and my go to (if you couldn't tell). I will say this however, you still have to be careful! Some wine has added flavors, and some are aged in barrels that contain gluten. Make sure you are careful with what you are drinking but enjoy it! Go ahead and pop that cork because you should be celebrating the fact that you can drink way more than you thought you could!

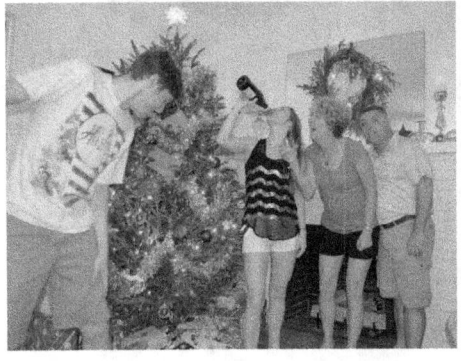

Photo: Christmas time in the Yancy household. Have I mentioned that I love wine? I also introduced my mom to wine, and my dad is standing there like "someone save me" and of course my brother photo bombing since he refused to take the photo with us. This... is an awesome photo!

# TACOS!!!

You don't know it yet, but I am about to blow your mind with some serious taco mayhem! I have mentioned tacos a few times throughout the book but I have not mentioned them enough! When I was in college I found new ways to cook tacos and I found a new appreciation for tacos! I have also noticed that all of the little taco shops around here in my part of town are the best places to go eat! I look forward to the Mexican tacos and I will never be able to make anything near as good as those are. BUT, don't fret the taco ideas are coming! Instead of giving you a bunch of recipes and becoming a typical recipe book, I left a lot of the taco making up to your imagination. Also, have you heard of Pinterest yet? That is the way to go when you need any recipe ideas, I mean seriously, they have everything! (If you can get past all of the wedding and home improvement ideas.)

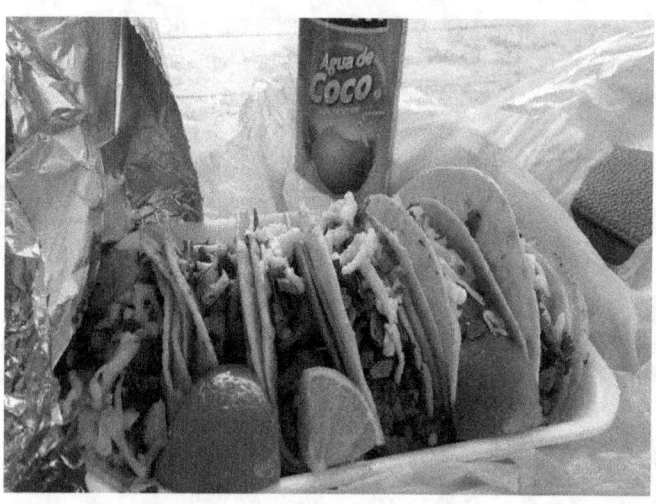

So, without further ado, I would like to introduce you to the great and wonderful taco ingredient list that you get to pick and chose from, to make the perfect taco! Here is how it works! Pick a protein from the top taco, and then choose all of your toppings from the bottom taco. Or, be adventurous and add all of the proteins with one topping. Mix and match, come up with your own combinations. Pull out the grill and aluminum foil and get ready to make your neighborhood smell like some seriously delicious tacos!

*Warning: This may lead to unwanted neighbors knocking on the door wondering what that fantastic smell is!* **ENJOY!**

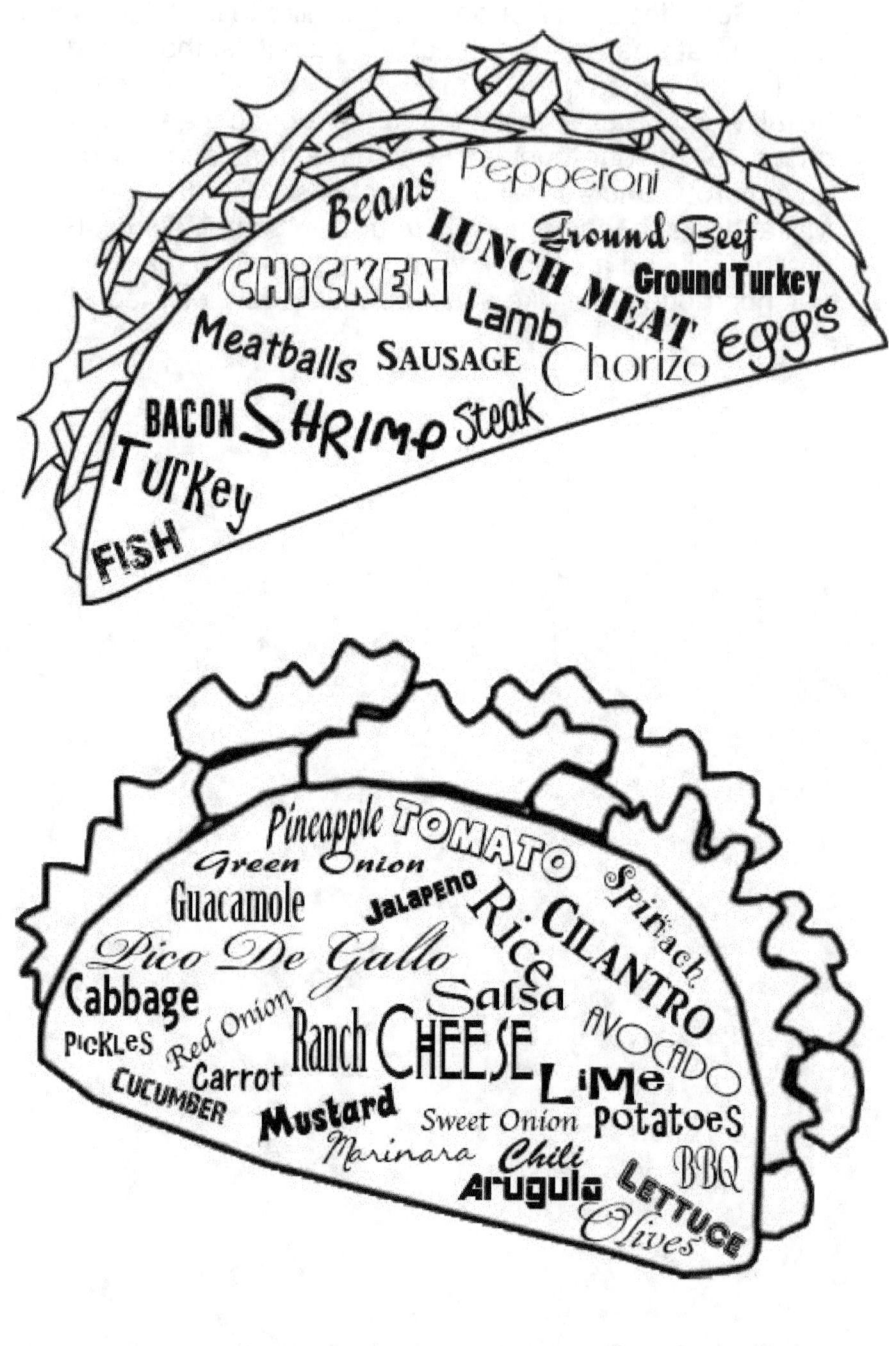

# REFERENCES

# WHOLE30.com

-Visit the website and purchase the book! Even if you choose not to do the
Whole 30 (which I completely understand) It is an awesome book to read and learn about the way your body works.

# Soverign Silver

https://www.natural-immunogenics.com/silver-101/
-This is one of the "medicines" I listed under my cabinet. Silver is not a medicine but it is a great product that can be used for more than you would imagine! If you are curious about what it is and how it helps there is a ton of information on their website that would lead you to understand all of the application of their product!

# Urban Tastebud

http://urbantastebud.com/category/gluten-free-2/
-This website is designed to make things even more easy than you thought they already were! It introduces new products, restaurants, and even more specifically the gluten free items you are allowed to eat and drink! Some of the gems I have found on their site are Halloween candy and alcohol lists that are GF!

# Pinterest

https://www.pinterest.com
-Only the greatest website for ideas ever! Check it out for cooking, cleaning, eating out, products, remedies, and other random things that you didn't know that you need.

# Celiac.org

-Super great information and an awesome way to dive in and learn more!

# Amazon.com
# Bobsredmill.com
# Wholefoodsmarket.com
# Celiacandthebeast.com
# Verywell.com
# Findmeglutenfree.com

# RESOURCES

# PLACES TO SHOP FOR GF ITEMS WITHOUT BREAKING THE BANK!

## In Store:
Big Lots (I was amazed at the amount of inventory they had!)
Fred Meyer
Kroger
Local City Market
Publix (Items listed online)
Trader Joe's (Items listed online)
Walmart (few items but still some available!)
Whole Foods

## Online:
The Gluten-Free Mall
Glutenfree.com
Free From Market

# PLACES TO EAT IN ORLANDO!!!

Hot Krust Panini Kitchen, (407) 355-7768
Nile Ethiopian Restaurant, (407) 354-0026
Raglan Road Irish Pub, (407) 938-0300
Dandelion Communitea Cafe, (407) 362-1864
Cooper's Hawk Winery & Restaurant, (407) 374-2464
Noodles and Rice, (407) 895-8833
Hawkers Asian Street Fare, (407) 237-0606
Smallcakes, (407) 681-7501
Le Macaron (321) 295-7958

**Make sure to call ahead and ask if gluten free options are available and make sure that they know you are coming at least an hour ahead of time!**

# ACKNOWLEDGMENTS

I have written the book about poop, which seems simple enough however, I can not say that it was an easy task. Actually, it has been a long process and I have spent many hours hiding behind closed bathroom doors, and curled up in bed or adding my imprint to the couch. All of that being said, I have a few people to say thanks to and not in any specific order!

I have already said thanks to my mother Lorri, my father Kevin, my brother Matt, and my grandma Carol, but I do not think that I can say it enough! They may not have believed me at first, but they surely made things so much easier and were very accommodating when I was laying on the floor passed out! And not to mention needing help with being fed and such. Oh, and always making light of a situation that felt like the world was collapsing on my head. There have been so many changes in the Yancy household! There are way more gluten free meals and eating out is not only stressful for me, but also for my family and it makes it easier to choose where we are going to eat out. I seriously have no words to tell you all how thankful I am for you being there and being a solid foundation for me.

To my other mother Nicki Watts who really isn' t a mother at all! However, she has all but adopted me and that is saying the absolute least. I can always expect that if she is at the supermarket, I will receive photos of new GF products, or she will show up on the doorstep with whatever else she has found! Including but not limited to, books, cereal, candy, cheese puffs, music (for my days when I am down), t-shirts, tea, and more. Not only will she surprise me with random odds and ends, she also finds ways to make me feel better when I am sad or sick.

To my Family whom I have not yet mentioned, you stay curious and always ask how I am doing. You may not see it when I am feeling poorly, but on the good days, I thoroughly enjoy being surrounded by you. The support you offer, means more than you could possibly imagine.

My dear friend Madison McDonald, you have been a true role model to me through this journey! Not only did you teach me how to stay positive when things just seem to be crashing down around you. You also led me into a habit of spending more time in prayer. You have been a low maintenance friend (because we both understand when the other bails), you continue to be a great deal of moral support and you are an all around amazing lady! Also, can we have a wine date soon?

To my friends and adopted family members (friends that are around as much if not more than family) you are the best! You bake cookies, send me recipes, and let me vent when I am convinced that I am dying from a gluten attack. When I feel like I can not talk to anyone else about my pain... I come to you! I actually feel sort of sorry for you all because I know I bail on plans so much but you totally understand and that is what makes you so unique and special to me!

And last, but definitely not least, to the special man in my life who not only steals all of my gluten free food and tells me (without filter) how he loves or hates it, but also makes it a point to make sure I am feeling well and eating reputable food. Your support means the world to me even if I don' t always show it! Sorry for ruining you with my inability to talk " like a lady" when I have been glutened. Thanks for allowing me to fill up your belly with gluten free treats! You make for a great test dummy my dear!

# NOTES